The Art of
NATURAL
CLEANING

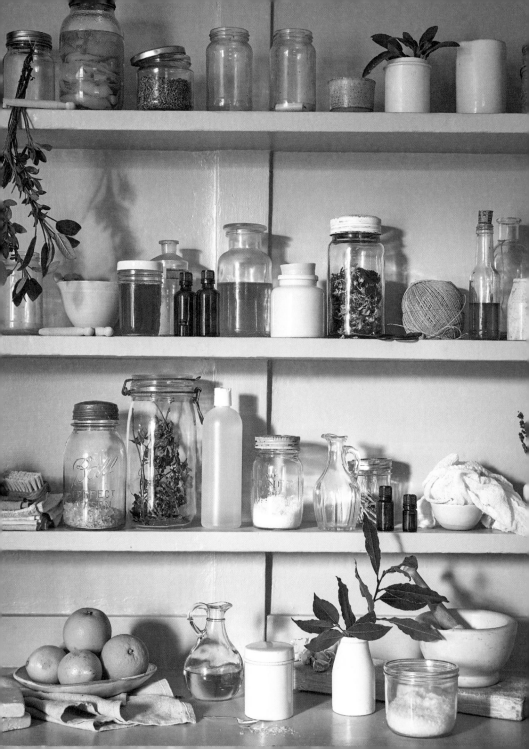

The Art of
NATURAL
CLEANING

Tips and techniques for a
chemical-free, sparkling home

Rebecca Sullivan

photography by Nassima Rothacker

Kyle Books

For the Clean Queen herself, my mum.

An Hachette UK Company
www.hachette.co.uk

First published in Great Britain in 2018 by
Kyle Books, an imprint of Kyle Cathie Limited
Carmelite House, 50 Victoria Embankment
London EC4Y 0DZ
www.kylebooks.co.uk

10 9 8 7 6 5 4 3

ISBN 978 0 85783 475 1

Text © 2018 Rebecca Sullivan
Design © 2018 Kyle Books
Photographs © 2018 Nassima Rothacker
Illustrations © 2018 Chrissy Lau

Distributed in the US by Hachette Book Group,
1290 Avenue of the Americas, 4th and 5th Floors,
New York, NY 10104

Distributed in Canada by Canadian Manda
Group, 664 Annette St.,
Toronto, Ontario,
Canada, M6S 2C8

Project Editor: Tara O'Sullivan
Copy Editor: Anne Sheasby
Editorial Assistant: Sarah Kyle
Designer: Laura Woussen
Photographer: Nassima Rothacker
Illustrator: Chrissy Lau
Stylists: Rebecca Sullivan and Rachel de Thample
Prop Stylist: Agathe Gits
Production: Lisa Pinnell

A Cataloguing in Publication record for this title is
available from the British Library.

Printed and bound in Europe

The information and advice contained in this
book are intended as a general guide to using
plants and are not specific to individuals or their
particular circumstances. Many plant substances,
whether sold as foods or as medicines and used
externally or internally, can cause an allergic
reaction in some people. Neither the author nor
the publishers can be held responsible for claims
arising from the inappropriate use of any remedy
or healing regime. Do not attempt self-diagnosis
or self-treatment for serious or long-term conditions
before consulting a medical professional or
qualified practitioner. Do not undertake any self-
treatment while taking other prescribed drugs or
receiving therapy without first seeking professional
guidance. Always seek medical advice if any
symptoms persist.

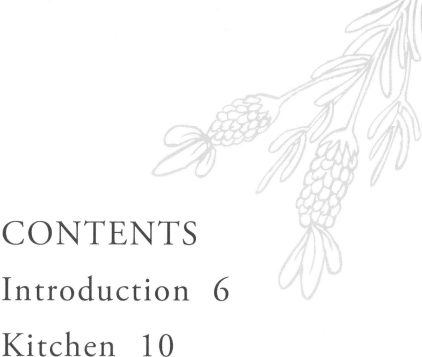

CONTENTS

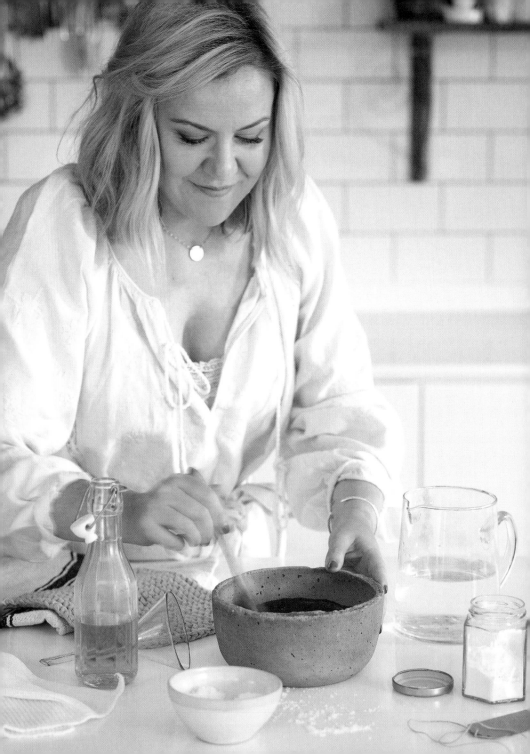

Introduction

Cleaning can be a bore. No doubt about it. Growing up, my mum kept an immaculate house (she still does), and as a kid it was more than irritating being constantly nagged to pick up after ourselves by the 'clean queen' as my brothers and I would call her (behind her back, of course). Nowadays, my house is clean. Not sterile, but clean. My bedroom, the only exception, is, from time to time, a mess (not unclean, but a mess). There is a difference between being a bit of a mess and being unclean. And there is a massive difference between being clean and being sterile.

I hate sterility. It was cleaning products that first set me on my natural home path. I remember cleaning my oven, which is used frequently, and coughing so much that it stopped me in my tracks. I just immediately knew it was toxic and checked the back label. I had no idea what any of the ingredients were or meant, and so that particular product and all the other bottles like it under my sink went in the bin. That, plus the fact that my nan, my muse and the reason for my work and creation of the Granny Skills Movement, still uses four things (well five) to clean her house. Bicarbonate of soda, lemon, vinegar, salt and elbow grease. And it works. Not only do they work, her homemade cleaning products are also all completely natural and edible – not that I would encourage anyone to eat any of them. But it makes me utterly comfortable in having them in my home. Because remember, if it's being sprayed in your home, it's going to end up in your body one way or another.

I am not perfect at this stuff by any means and I hope I don't sound like too much of a bore in saying any of this, but we are the only ones that have control over our bodies and our homes. We can make the choice to go chemical-free, and in doing so we take back control. We help the planet. We help our health and we help our wallets. Let's not forget that! Let's stop saying we don't have time to do this. Most of the recipes in this book take seconds and minutes, not hours, to make. We can change our priorities at the flick of a switch (the off one on our mobile phones is a good start!).

Another thing that bothers me is when you go into a café and see someone scrubbing everything in sight with anti-bacterial wipes, and the constant over-use of super toxic hand sanitisers. There is such a thing as killing good bacteria, too. We have all gone crazy. Being sterile is NOT good for us (unless you work in a hospital). We need dirt, we need bugs and we all need to stop being so intense. A clean home is great, a sterile one can actually be unhealthy.

So, it's time to detox the cupboards and top up with a few essentials. I would always suggest making these recipes in small batches as you need them rather than large batches. They are best used fresh as they don't contain any non-natural preservatives.

SHOPPING LIST
- Vinegar – white, wine and apple cider.
- Salt – an array of different salts – coarse salt makes a great scourer.
- Bicarbonate of soda – literally your new bestie.
- Lemons and oranges.
- Olive oil – you have it anyway.
- Castile soap – have it on hand for many of these recipes.
- Essential oils – these are an investment, but will last a long time and change your home for the better.

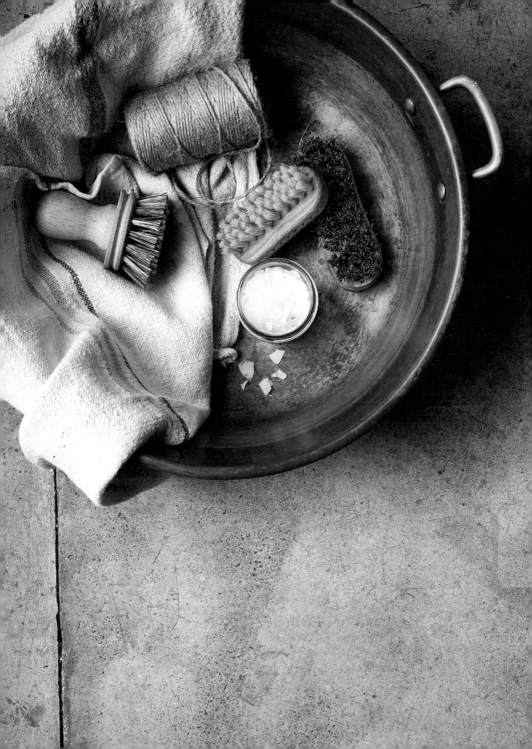

Chapter One
kitchen

Orange all-round kitchen spray

This will clean and sterilise all surfaces – kitchen and bathroom – and leave everything smelling delicious. Also a fab way to use up the orange peels that often get discarded and wasted.

MAKES 400ML

peel from 4 oranges
200ml white vinegar

500ml glass jar
recycled spray bottle

Tightly pack the orange peel into a glass jar and cover with the white vinegar. Put the lid on, and then leave to stand for 4 weeks. Gently shake the jar occasionally during this period.

Strain the vinegar into a spray bottle and top up with an equal amount of water; shake briefly to combine. Spray directly onto surfaces and wipe with a damp cloth. This will keep indefinitely.

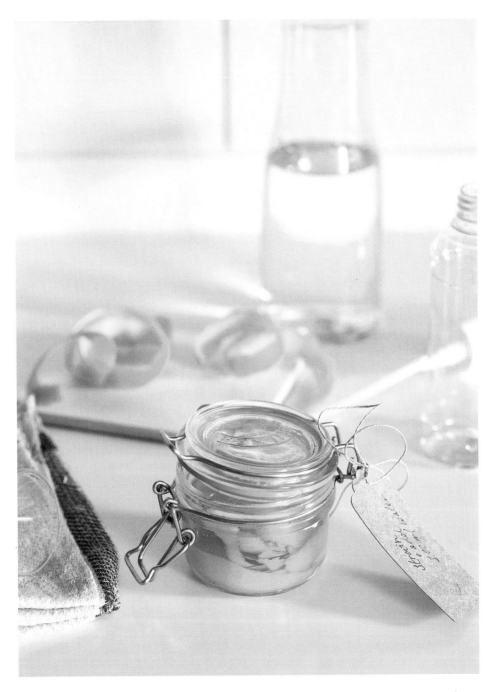

Eco cloths & dusters

Dish cloths. Dusting cloths. All of the various cloths we can buy. They make cleaning easy because when they get all gross and too dirty, we can just dispose of them in the rubbish if we wish. But please don't do this!!! They just contribute to landfill. Instead of buying new cloths, why not reinvent other items that have already served their first purpose?

Use cut up old t-shirts or shirts as dusting or general cleaning cloths. Use old tea towels cut into squares as dishcloths. Towels cut into squares make great dishwashing cloths too, or use them as facecloths or flannels, and if you can crochet, then crochet some squares and use them for the dishes. Whichever of these you use, they can all then be thrown in the washing machine and used over and over again.

For a feather duster, literally start to gather old feathers, and once you have a large enough bunch, first disinfect the feathers by soaking them in some warm water with a little lemon juice and white vinegar added, then rinse and dry in the sun. Tie the base of the feathers to a long stick with some twine to hold them in place, and voilà.

Salt scourer

Salt. My nan always told me it was magic and she was right. Not only fantastic for cooking and skin care, the salt shaker can be useful for cleaning too.

FOR EACH USE

coarse salt

½ a lemon (optional)

jar with a lid

Fill an old jam jar with really coarse salt. Poke holes in the jar lid. Now every time you have a stubborn stain on a worktop, in the oven or in a saucepan, sprinkle some salt onto the surface, then add a tiny bit of water or, better still, a squeeze of lemon juice. Use the cut side of the lemon (if using) face down, or a cloth and scour away. Rinse with water.

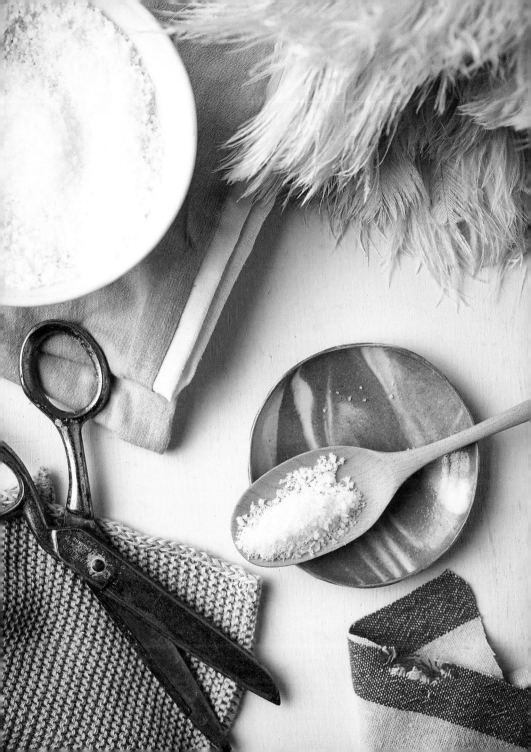

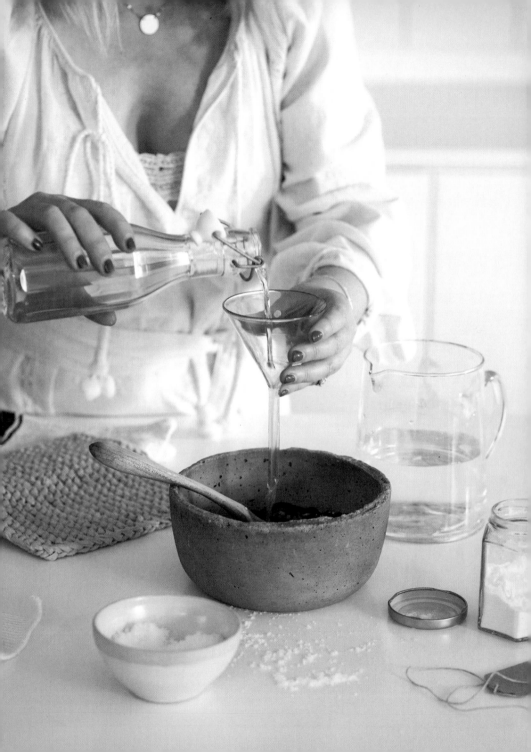

Oven cleaner

There is nothing worse than the smell of chemical oven spray. It literally makes you cough, so you can only imagine what is in it. Sure it's quick and easy, but with a tiny bit of elbow grease and patience, you can have a chemical-free, clean oven.

MAKES ENOUGH
FOR A SINGLE USE

60g bicarbonate of soda
60ml white vinegar
coarse salt

spray bottle

Place the bicarbonate of soda in a small bowl and add a little cold water at a time, mixing until it forms a paste. Wearing rubber gloves, take a cloth and rub the paste over the entire surface of your cold oven. Depending on the size of your oven, you may need to make a little more. Leave for 12 hours to work its magic.

After that time, wipe all of the surfaces with kitchen paper and discard. Put the vinegar in a spray bottle and spritz all the surfaces of your oven. Use salt as a scourer for any stubborn stains by sprinkling it directly onto the cloth, scrubbing, then rinsing using a cloth and some warm water to continue to remove all of the residue. Give all the surfaces a final wipe down with clean warm water and leave to dry.

If you only try one recipe in this book, make it this one and free yourself from chemical oven cleaner forever!

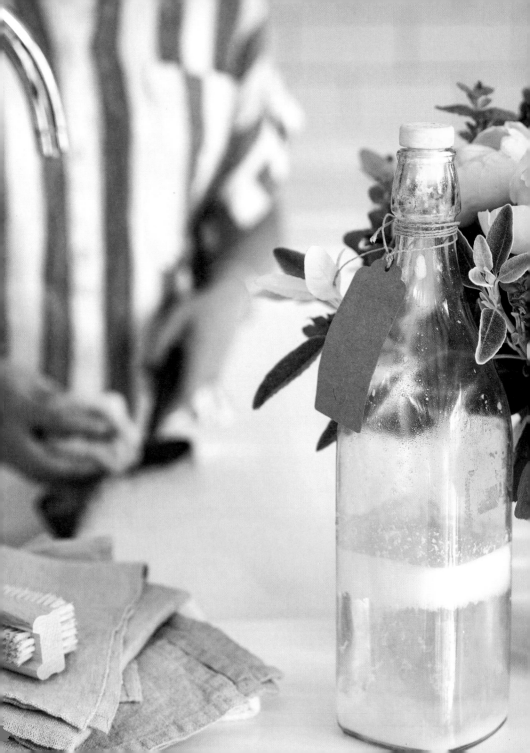

Washing-up liquid

This washing-up liquid will not foam and bubble like you'll be used to, but that is normally because something artificial has been added to the liquid. So if you want clean dishes, it will clean them, but don't freak out if there are no or few bubbles.

MAKES 525ML

2 tablespoons bicarbonate of soda
3 tablespoons liquid castile soap
450ml boiled water
15 drops of lemon essential oil
a few slices of fresh lemon

recycled storage/squirty bottle

Put the bicarbonate of soda and soap in a medium bowl and pour over the boiling water. Mix until it is all combined. Leave the mixture to cool completely, then pour into a storage bottle (something easy to use like a squirty bottle, and a recycled one is great). Add the essential oil and lemon slices, then shake and store under the sink.

When using, add a little at a time to hot water, depending on how soapy you like the water to wash your dishes. Also refresh the lemon slices from time to time as they will get a little mouldy if left for too long (not the dangerous kind of mould, but just be aware of it and make another batch if it happens). This will keep for about a year.

Hand wash

This can either be a foaming hand wash or a liquid one, but it works better in a foaming bottle, which you can buy online. Just by adding essential oils to your liking, you can make a hand soap just like the ones in the bathrooms at fancy hotels – only a million times cheaper and a million times more luxurious.

MAKES 330ML

300ml filtered water (or more, depending on the size of the bottle you buy)

2 tablespoons liquid castile soap

a few drops of olive or nut oil

6–8 drops of your favourite essential oil (for smell) – lavender, tea tree and eucalyptus are naturally antibacterial so perfect for this

foaming bottle/soap dispenser

Fill your foaming bottle with the filtered water, leaving about 2.5cm of space for the other ingredients. Now add the liquid soap and olive or nut oil, then finish with the essential oil. Stir or swirl gently to combine and put on the lid. Use as required.

This will last for a few months. I prefer to make this kind of thing in small batches and more frequently.

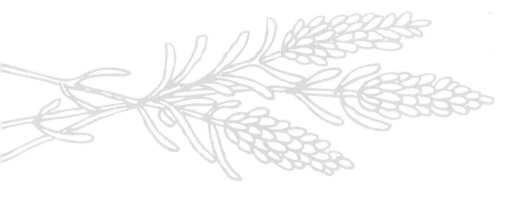

Dishwasher detergent

I'm not going to lie. This recipe has been the hardest to get right because I didn't want to add shop-bought additions. I think the addition of lemon halves and vinegar gets it pretty close to shop-bought dishwasher tablets. But a polish of your glasses will still be needed at times.

MAKES 20 APPLICATIONS

For the detergent

250g salt
500g bicarbonate of soda

For each wash

60ml white vinegar
1 lemon, cut in half

large glass jar with a lid

To make the detergent, mix the salt and bicarbonate of soda together in a bowl, then transfer to a large glass jar to store.

When it's time to do a load of dishes, add 2 tablespoons of the dry detergent mix to the tablet compartment in your dishwasher and the vinegar to the rinse section. Firmly wedge the lemon halves in the dishwasher, either in the cutlery holder or somewhere where they won't fly about. Put your wash on as normal.

The jar of dry detergent mix will keep in a cool, dry place for up to 6 months.

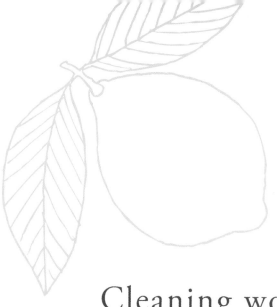

Cleaning wooden chopping boards

A quick way to gross you out would be to tell you that there is 200 times more bacteria living on your chopping board than your toilet seat. Gross I know but if cleaned properly then it's really not that gross. I use this method when I use my board for anything like veggies or meat (not for bread). Salt, lemon and sunshine are all your board needs to keep it fresh and clean.

FOR EACH USE

salt, any is fine but coarse is good
for grit and stains
1 lemon, cut in half

Sprinkle the chopping board(s) with salt, then squeeze over some lemon juice. Scrub the board(s) using the cut sides of the lemon halves as scourers. Rinse in hot water and put outside in the sunshine to dry.

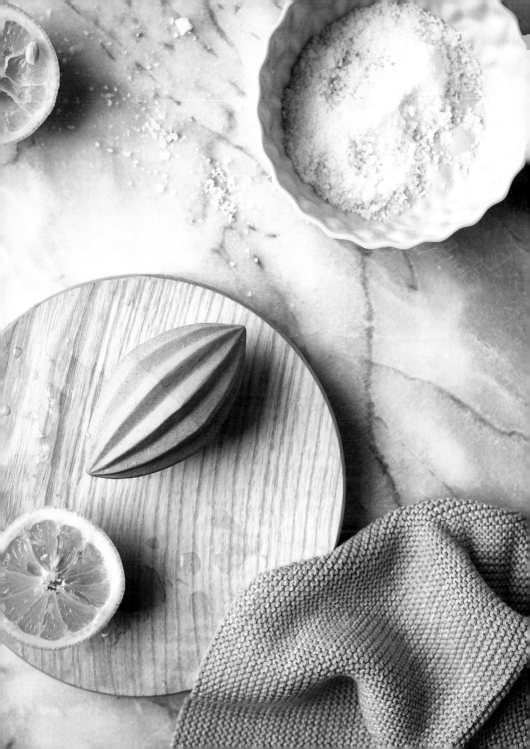

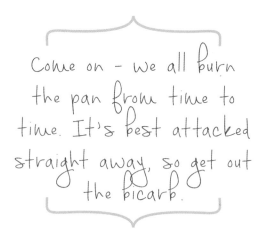

Come on - we all burn the pan from time to time. It's best attacked straight away, so get out the bicarb.

Whoops I burnt the pan (again)

We are all guilty of the odd burnt pan now and again. And who has the time or inclination to scrub for hours? None of us. Nor do any of us really want to use the cut-throat poisons that remove the burnt-on food with one swift wipe (there is a reason for that). Try this instead. Guilt-free pan cleaning.

FOR EACH USE
generous sprinkle of bicarbonate of soda
splash of white vinegar

Take your burnt pan. Sprinkle it generously with bicarbonate of soda and leave overnight. The next day, place the pan on your hob. Add a splash of vinegar and a little water.

Bring to the boil, then simmer gently for a couple of minutes. Turn the heat off, discard the liquid, and you should now be able to remove any burnt bits with warm water and a cloth. Rinse and dry.

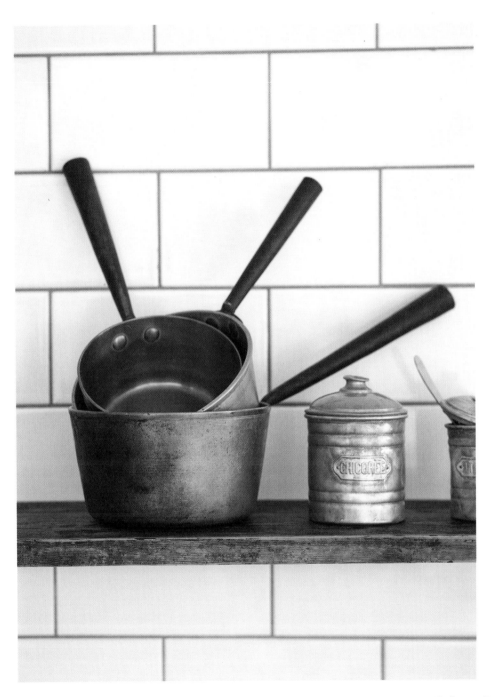

Chapter Two

wardrobe
& laundry

Moth balls

There is nothing more irritating than pulling out your favourite sweater at the beginning of winter to find it has holes in it, having been munched on by the moths. Shop-bought moth repellents can be full of nasties, such as camphor and dichlorobenzene, and often smell awful. These handmade ones are not nasty at all and will also make your clothes smell delightful. In short, the moths hate these smells and should stay well away from your cashmere.

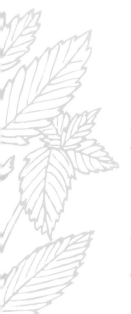

MAKES 2

an old pair of tights or stockings
or some old thin muslin
2 cotton wool balls
ribbon or twine

choose from one of the following
dried herb (and fruit/spice)
mixtures

* **½ handful of rosemary and**
  ½ handful of peppermint or
  garden mint
* **½ handful of lavender and ½**
  handful of rosemary
* **⅓ handful each of dried citrus**
  peel, broken-up cinnamon stick
  and lavender
* **some dried rose petals for an**
  extra appealing scent (optional)
* **a few drops of essential oils to**
  match the scents of the herbs
  chosen above

Cut off the legs of your stockings or tights – you only need the foot part for this. Mix your chosen herbs together, adding some dried rose petals to the mix, if you like. Add the drops of essential oils to the cotton wool balls.

Fill each stocking/tight foot with a cotton wool ball and half of the herb mix, or use two squares of the muslin measuring about 15cm x 15cm. Tie a knot in the top of each, then finish with a piece of ribbon or twine. Place in your drawer, give each sachet a scrunch and hey presto!

Scrunch to release the oils every so often (about once a month) to keep the moths at bay. Replace every couple of months with a fresh sachet.

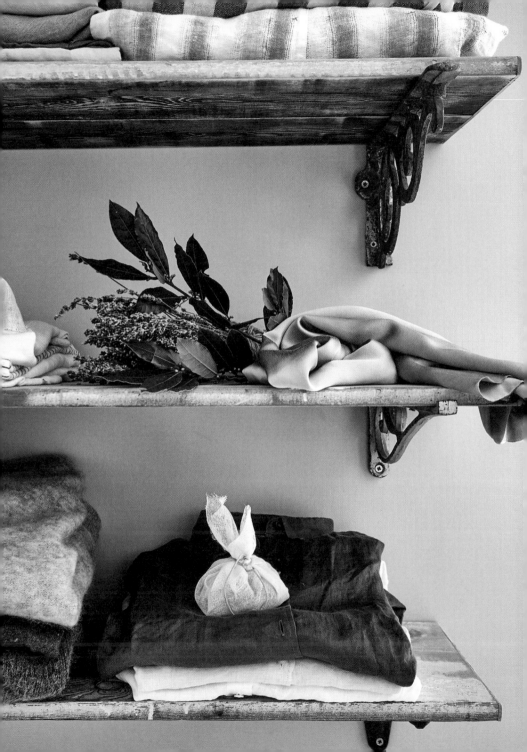

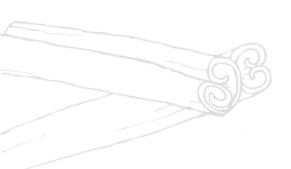

Linen sachets

These remind me of my great-grandmother's knickers drawer. Not sure how I know this, but I am pretty certain it comes from always rummaging through her jewellery boxes and drawers looking for treasures, and laughing at her gigantic(ish) lady briefs. Her drawers smelt like lavender. In fact, her entire body smelt of it. She used lavender on everything because she was an insomniac and lavender helped a little. She bathed in it, sipped it, used it in talc. Literally everything. The smell of it brings a massive smile to my face and a flutter in my heart.

MAKES 1 LINEN SACHET

1 teaspoon dried lavender

1 teaspoon dried rose petals

1 cinnamon stick, broken into pieces

1 dried orange slice or fresh peel

1 teaspoon dried peppermint

15cm square piece of muslin or soft cotton cloth

piece of twine

Mix all the ingredients together in a small bowl, then place in the centre of the piece of muslin or cotton cloth. Gather the cloth around the filling and tie with twine.

Place the sachet in a drawer, and squish it every now and then to release the scents. Replace every couple of months.

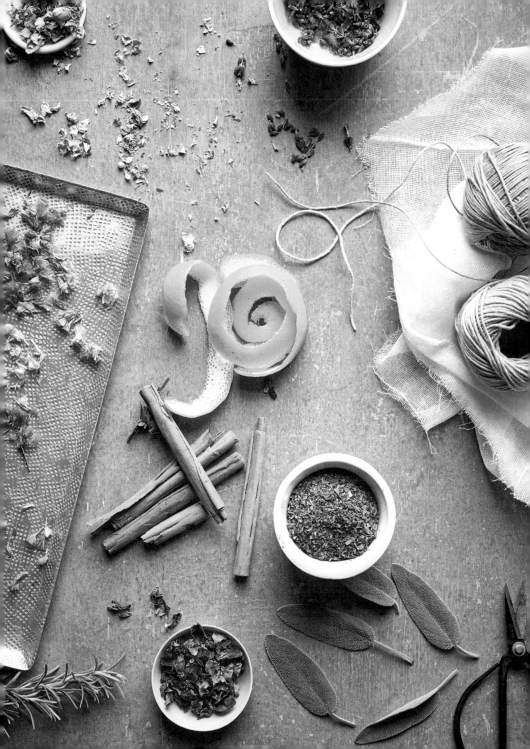

Drawer liners

These are similar to the linen sachets on page 30, but are scented liners rather than sachets. They fit nicely into a drawer and every time you open it a little waft of pretty scent will make you smile.

MAKES 1 DRAWER LINER

a combination of dried ingredients such as rose petals, cinnamon sticks (broken into pieces), lavender, peppermint, dried citrus, rosemary and thyme – small handful of each.

double-sided Velcro® (or other fabric hook-and-loop fastener)
an old pillowcase per drawer (cotton or linen is best)

Attach two sets of double-sided Velcro® to the inside of the pillow case, so that the case can be divided into three compartments. This will help you to keep the ingredients evenly dispersed throughout the case.

Mix up the dried ingredients of your choice and place inside the pillow case, spreading them out evenly. Now secure the Velcro® strips so that the pillow case has three filled pockets.

If you wish, you can put more Velcro® strips on the back of the pillow case, with corresponding strips on the base of the drawer itself, to hold the liner in place in your drawer.

Place the liner into your drawer, and press down on it every now and then to release the scents. Replace every couple of months.

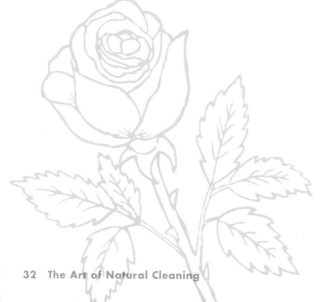

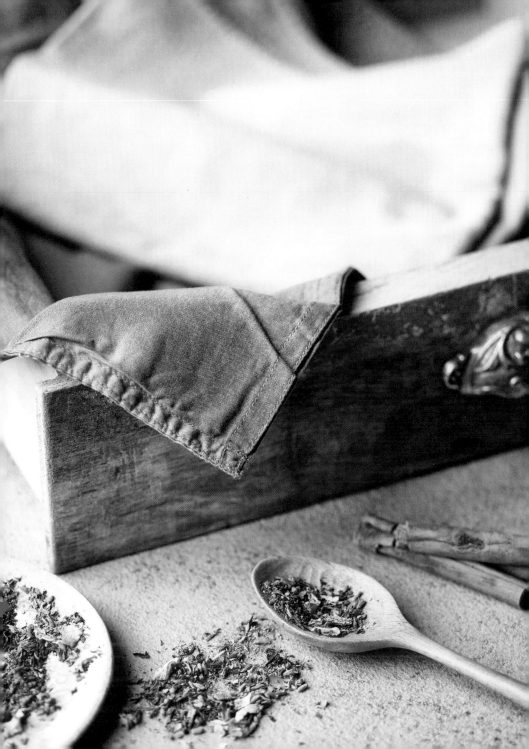

Shoe polish

Shiny shoes remind me of my dad. These days he is more of a steel-cap boots kind of man, but I remember seeing many a photo of him in his navy days with sparkling clean black shoes. It also makes me chuckle a little as my brothers went to a private school and they had to polish their shoes all the time. I went to a public school and didn't have to. Suckers.

MAKES 50G

2 tablespoons beeswax
2 tablespoons olive or nut oil
2 tablespoons cocoa butter

small recycled tin
clean, dry cloth

Always use this polish on clean, dry shoes. It is for leather shoes only and will stain suede.

Melt all the ingredients together in a double boiler over a low heat. If you don't have a double boiler, use a heatproof bowl set over a pan of barely simmering water (making sure the bottom of the bowl doesn't touch the water underneath).

Pour the melted mixture into a small recycled tin and leave it to cool and harden, before putting the lid on and storing until ready to use. Use on clean leather surfaces.

Clean your shoes with either a bristle brush or a wet cloth, then leave to dry completely. Polish your shoes in the usual way with a clean, dry cloth and this polish. The beeswax acts as a leather protector on your shoes. This polish will keep for up to a year.

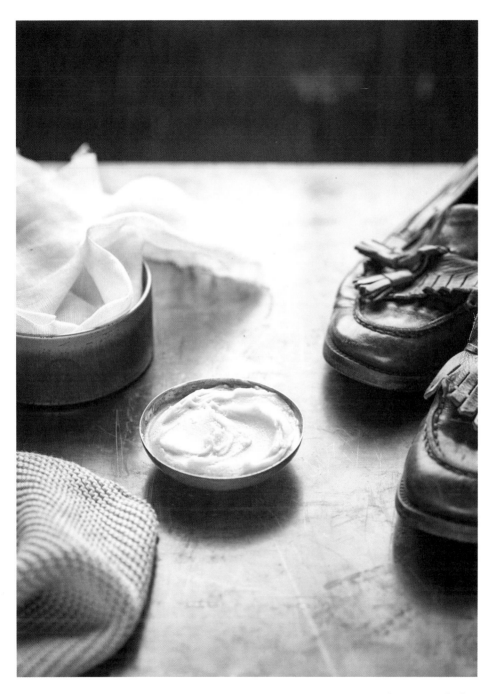

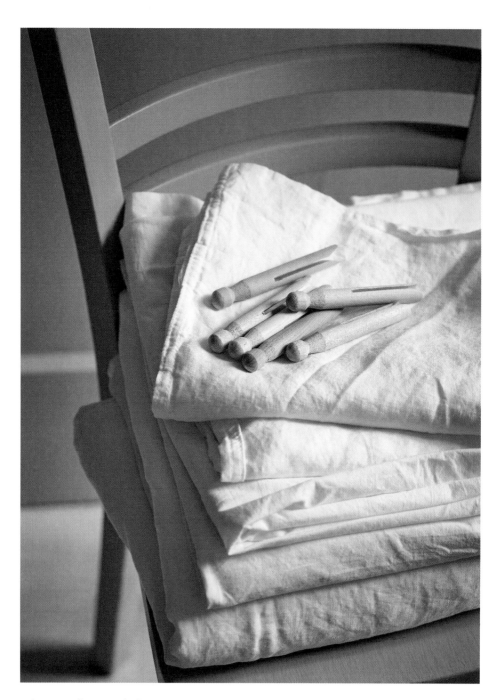

Washing powder

My partner, Damien, is an obsessive washer of clothes. I am more of a 'if it ain't dirty, don't wash it' kind of girl. I hate to a) waste water, and b) deteriorate my clothes. Damien has come round a little, but at least using this washing powder I don't feel as bad about what's going into the waste water.

MAKES 650G

100–150g bar of natural soap (real soap, such as Dr Bronner's or Castile – not glycerine-filled)
250g bicarbonate of soda
250g natural washing soda (soda crystals)
10 drops of lemon or orange essential oil

Chop or grate the soap into small pieces. Put all of the ingredients into a food processor and blitz to a fine powder. Let the mixture settle before opening the lid as the particles are fine. Transfer to an airtight container to store. This will last for up to a few months, but it's best made more frequently in small batches.

Use between 1–3 tablespoons per wash, depending on how dirty your clothes are.

Fabric softener

This will leave your towels fluffy and your undies silky, your sheets like clouds and your dresses all floaty.

MAKES 1.9 LITRES
(about 30 applications)

1 litre filtered water
400ml natural hair conditioner
500ml apple cider vinegar
20 drops of lavender essential oil or a mix of your favourites

recycled airtight container or plastic bottle

Mix everything together in a recycled airtight container or plastic bottle. Shake before each use and use about 60ml per load of washing. If you like, you can add a teaspoon of eucalytpus or tea tree oil to your fabric softener dispenser to help with cleanliness.

This will keep for up to 6 months.

'DIY' orange oil

This is surprisingly easy to make and smells amazing. The perfect addition to your cleaning products.

MAKES ANYWHERE
BETWEEN 50–100ML

freshly peeled orange peel (enough to fill a 1 litre jar), cut into 2.5cm pieces

35cl bottle vodka (cheap is fine)

large jar with a lid

some muslin cloth or a paper coffee filter (even a new soft dishcloth is fine)

small sterilised jar for storage string

Line a tray with kitchen paper.

Use a few drops at a time in any recipe that calls for orange essential oil.

Spread out the orange peel on the tray, then leave to dry in a warm spot, away from direct sunlight, until really tough and hard. Around 2 days is usually about right depending on humidity. The smaller the pieces the faster they will dry.

Once dried, chop them into smaller pieces. Put the diced peel into a large ,clean glass jar. Now fill your sink with hot water and submerge the bottle of vodka for a minute or two to warm it. Pour enough vodka into the jar until it completely covers the orange peel.

Screw on the lid and shake the jar for 1–2 minutes. Now remember to do this a few times a day for 3 or more days.

Once ready, strain the vodka into a bowl using your cloth or a coffee filter. Do this by pouring the peel and vodka into the cloth or filter over a bowl, then tie it with some string and squeeze. Squeeze all of the liquid into the bowl. Cover the bowl with a clean tea towel. Leave it to stand in a cool place for a few more days. Once all the alcohol has evaporated, the leftover liquid will be your orange essential oil. Pour the concentrated orange oil into a sterilised small glass bottle or jar, close the lid, label and store in a cool, dark place for up to 6 months.

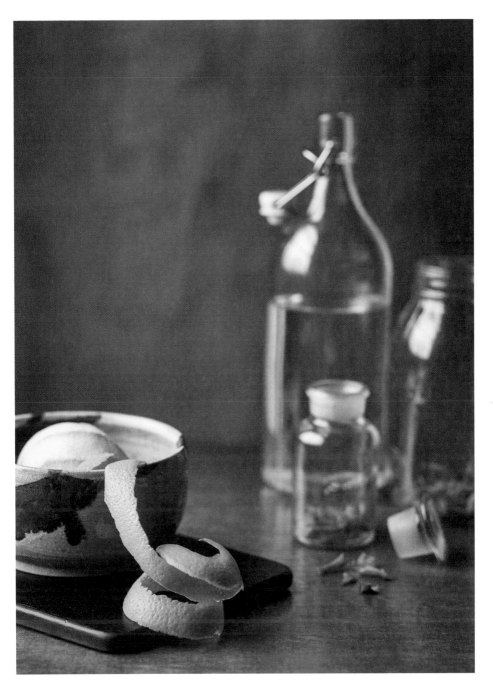

Chapter Three
bathroom

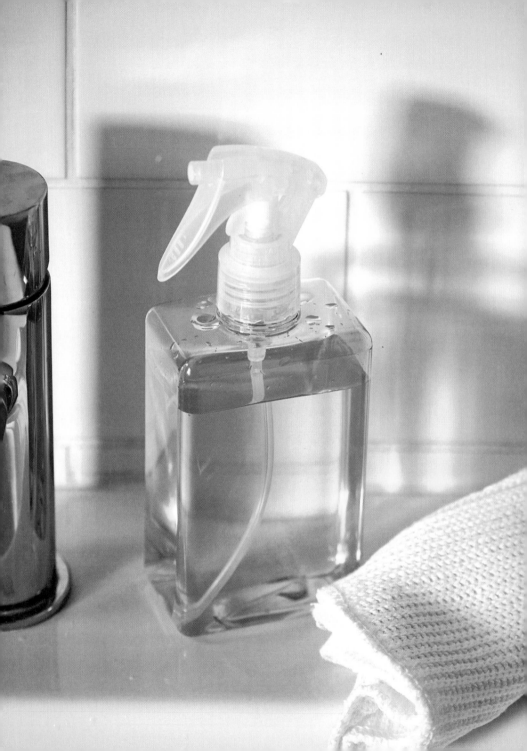

Bathroom cleaner

Streaky glass is a pain, just as much as cleaning the bathroom is. Keep this spray bottle to hand and every third day, give your shower and bath tub a spray and rinse. Then you won't have to scrub it every week. It will just stay clean.

MAKES 600ML

500ml warm water
30g bicarbonate of soda
50ml white vinegar

recycled spray bottle

Pour the warm water (not hot, just warm) into a bowl, then slowly pour in the bicarbonate of soda, stirring as you pour. Add the vinegar and stir to mix.

Pour into a recycled spray bottle, label and leave to cool. Store in a cool, dark place for up to 3 months.

Shake well before use and use as required. When using, spray onto the shower or bath surface, scrub if necessary, and then rinse with warm water to avoid streaks. It will . streak or form white marks if not rinsed thoroughly.

I keep a bottle of this in the shower so that every couple of days I can give everything a quick spray, wipe and rinse.

Toilet bombs

These are so cool. I prefer to make them without a mould, but you can do either. If you're not using a mould, you may find your mix is too dry, so just add a few drops of water until you can shape the mix into balls. Leave them to dry properly before storing. If they break, fret not, as they still do their job.

MAKES 10–12

250g bicarbonate of soda
80g citric acid
food colouring (optional)
dried flower petals, such as rose
    or lavender to decorate, slightly
    crushed (optional)
10 drops of rose essential oil
10 drops of lavender essential oil
5 drops of lemon essential oil

rubber gloves
cotton face mask
spray bottle
glass jar, for storage
ice cube trays or jelly molds

Wear rubber gloves and a face mask, not because the citric acid is a bad chemical, but it is strong and if it goes down your throat the wrong way you will cough. Mix the bicarbonate of soda and citric acid together in a glass bowl. Fill a spray bottle with some cold water and then very gradually spray water into the mix in the bowl, stirring as you go. You want to add just enough water (so hardly any) to make the ingredients stick together. You can add a few drops of food colouring or dried flower petals too, if you like.

Add the essential oils and continue mixing. Form the mixture into single-use sizes by pressing into small ball shapes or similar walnut-sized balls using your hands (or you can use individual moulds, such as ice cube trays, to shape the mixture). Place them on a tray and leave to dry overnight, then carefully transfer the bombs (popping them out of the moulds, if necessary) to a glass jar or other airtight container and close the lid. These will keep for up to 3 months.

To use, drop one into the toilet pan, leave it to dissolve and flush on the next use. Use as necessary, but no more than once a day.

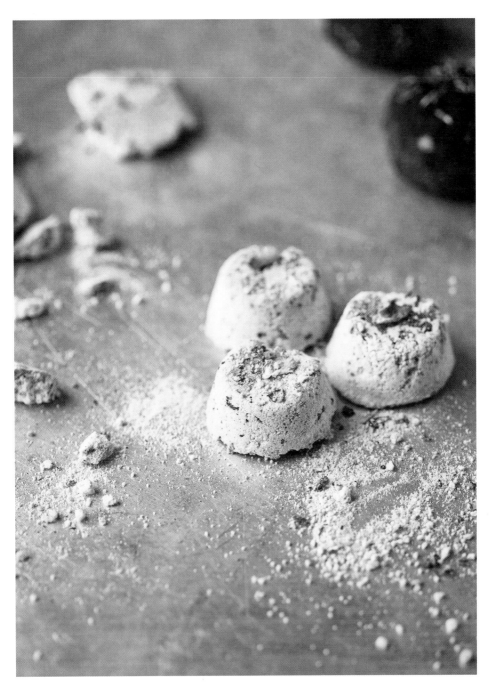

Handy wipes

Eek. When I think about poor baby's bottoms being scrubbed so frequently with baby wipes I get a little sad. These, however, make me happy. They are super natural and great for all of us, not just for mums and babies.

MAKES 50–100 WIPES

240ml witch hazel

1 tablespoon aloe vera gel

1 tablespoon raw organic coconut
  oil or nut oil

10 drops of lavender essential oil

10 drops of eucalyptus essential oil

1 roll of kitchen paper

1 medium-sized Tupperware or
  plastic container big enough to
  hold half a roll

Mix everything, except the kitchen paper, together in the Tupperware or plastic container. Using a sharp knife, carefully cut your roll of kitchen paper in half horizontally. Place half the roll (wrap and save the other half for the next batch), into the container, put the lid on and shake it.

Leave for 20 minutes, then pull out and discard the inner cardboard roll. Pull up a piece of the now-wet kitchen paper from the centre and put the lid back on. Use as required. These will keep fresh and moist in the closed container for up to 6 weeks.

For anti-bacterial wipes, follow the method above, instead using 240ml cold water, 75ml apple cider vinegar and 8 drops each of tea tree, eucaplyptus and lemon essential oils.

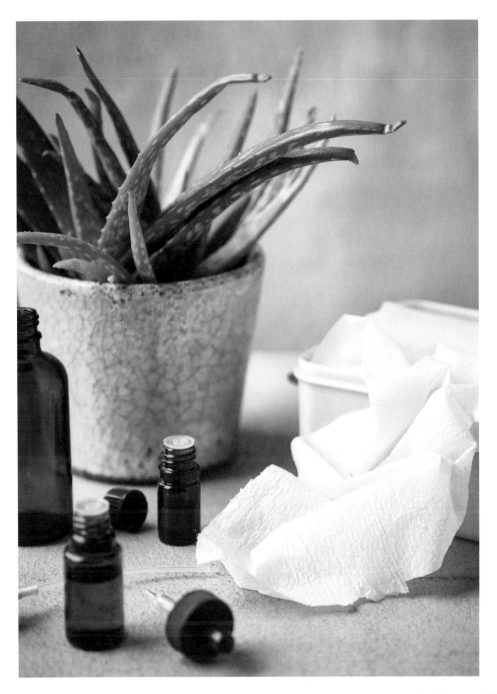

Chapter Four
scent

Odour Eaters

Smelly socks, smelly shoes, smelly rooms. Not all smells are created equal and not all smells are easily disguised with a room freshener or some perfume. Try to remove them first before refreshing the room. It works much better than trying to cover it up. These tips and tricks below will remove smells so you can then add the fragrance you want in the air.

- For your shoes – sprinkle bicarbonate of soda into them and leave them in the sun for the day. Hoover out when done.

- For the fridge – place a small dish of bicarbonate of soda on one of the shelves towards the back. Replace every month.

- For the home – place a small dish of used coffee grinds from the coffee pot in each room in a discreet place.

- For the toilet – sprinkle some bicarbonate of soda around the toilet pan and place a couple of lemon halves in the bowl. Leave to sit for a few hours, then discard the lemons and flush away the bicarb.

- For the washing machine – add a scoop of bicarbonate of soda to your next wash. Not only does it removes smells, it brightens clothes too.

- For your hands – if you've been handling garlic or fish, rub a cut lemon over your hands and rinse off.

- For your carpet – sprinkle the carpet with bicarbonate of soda and leave overnight. Hoover up the next day.

- For your rubbish bin – first, remove the bag if you use one, then sprinkle in some bicarbonate of soda every time you empty the bin. Every third or fourth time, rinse and put your bin out in the sunshine to dry. Sun is the best anti-bacterial cleanser you can get.

- For the sink – pour 6 tablespoons of bicarbonate of soda and 6 tablespoons of salt down the plughole, followed by a small pan or kettleful of boiling water. This is great for clogged drains too.

- For your sofa – if your sofa is one with zip covers, place bunches of dried lavender just inside the cushion covers (or in the scatter cushions on top), then each time you sit, a waft of lavender should come your way.

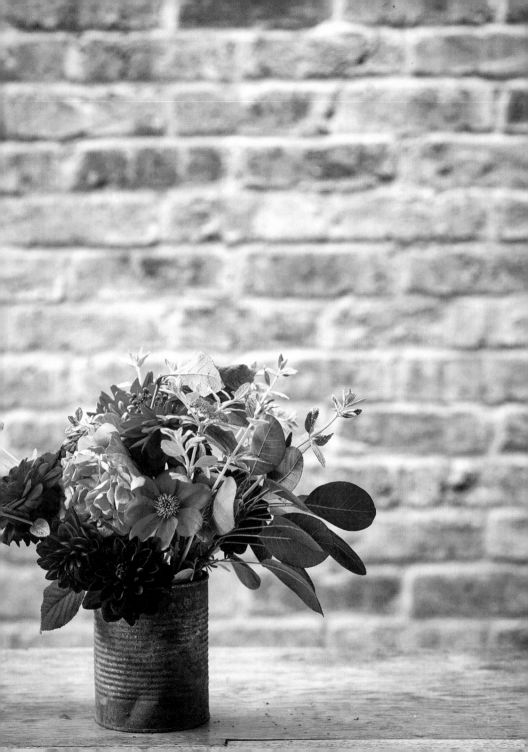

Diffuser

Diffusers remind me of super fancy bathrooms in really expensive restaurants. Well, guess what. This one costs under a fiver and you can make it smell like a real garden, not a fake and sickly coconuts on a beach kind of smell. Yuck. These are best made in small batches and used fresh.

MAKES 1 DIFFUSER

125–250ml carrier oil (such as extra virgin, fractionated coconut, avocado, apricot or nut oil)

20–40 drops of your chosen essential oil or a blend of essential oils of your choice

TRY:

Lemon and orange

Lavender and rose

Rosemary and thyme

Lemon and cinnamon

– the fun part is experimenting!

a pack of bamboo skewers (the ones you use for a barbecue)

an old jar or a small pretty vase or jug

Depending on how big your chosen vessel is (an old jar or a small pretty vase or jug is perfect), cut the skewers to be double the length of the height of the vessel. Remove the spiky ends so they look fancy (and no longer like barbecue skewers). Pour in the carrier oil and blend in your favourite essential oils until it smells just the way you like it.

Place a handful of the skewers in the vessel and leave them to soak for an hour. Remove the skewers, turn them upside down and return them to the vessel.

Position the vessel in your favourite place to impress, and voilà. Turn the skewers every now and then and top up the scented oil as needed.

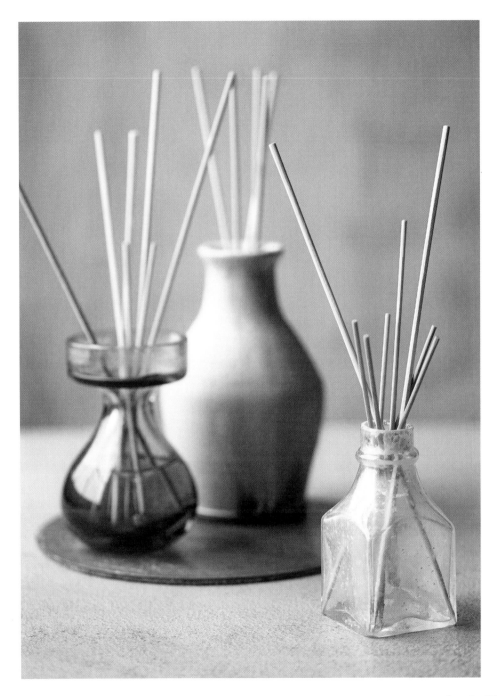

Herby floral burn sticks

Not just for hippies, these burn sticks are beautiful. They smell great and get rid of bad vibes in your home. Give them to your bestie for a pressie with a little crystal. OK, that's a little hippy. But I love hippies. You can use dried or fresh of any of the herbs or flowers listed below. If using fresh, you will need to hang and dry out the assembled burn sticks before use.

FOR EACH BURN STICK

a small bunch of one of the
   following:
sage or white sage leaves
cedar
pine
rosemary
lavender
roses

cotton twine

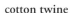

For each burn stick, bundle together your chosen herbs or flowers, keeping the stems together. Wind cotton twine quite tightly along its length (as though you are making a cigar or fat stick). If you are using fresh herbs, the twine will loosen as the herbs dry and shrink a bit. Now wind the twine back around the bundle in the other direction all along its length, crossing over the twine already on the bundle.

If you are using fresh herbs, hang the herb/flower burn sticks somewhere cool and dry and leave them to air-dry for a couple of weeks until completely dry. Dried herb/flower burn sticks can be used straightaway.

To burn, hold the stem/stalk end of the burn stick and light the other end until a flame gets going, then blow it out, place the burn stick in a small heatproof bowl or stand it up (stem/stalk-end down) in a heatproof vessel (such as a small vase, milk jug or pot) and let the smell waft about.

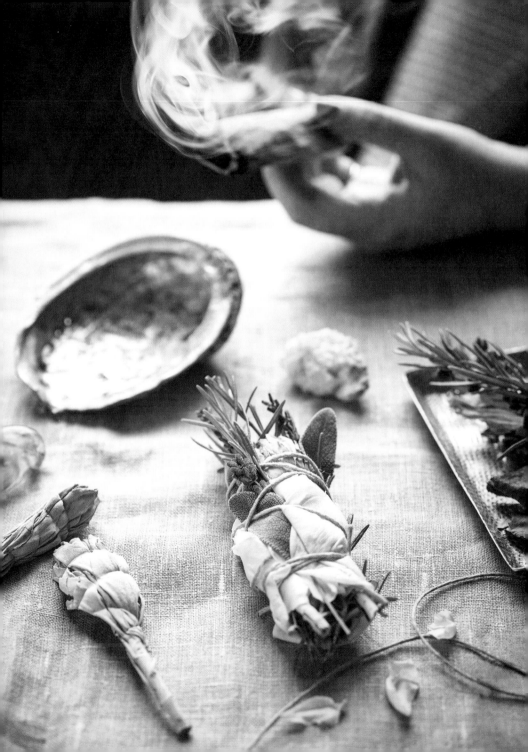

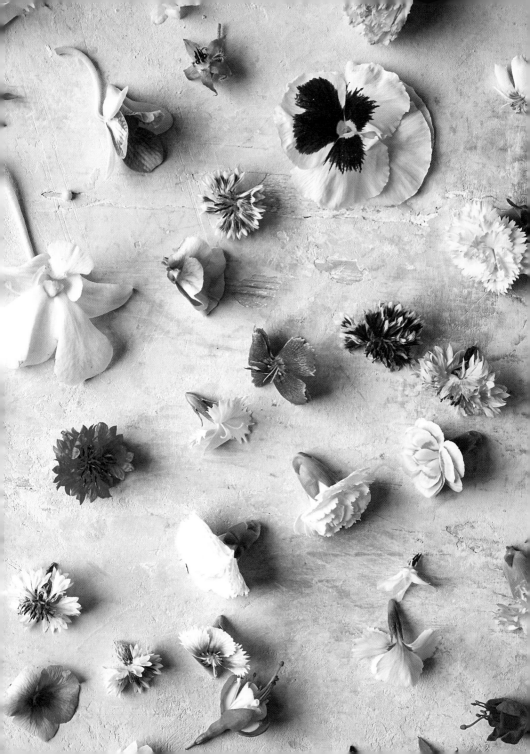

Potpourri

If the idea of a bowlful of potpourri is reminiscent of great aunt Mildred's house, or if lavender sachets are something for your grandma's knickers drawer, it's time to take a fresh look at something we have been doing since the dawn of time.

The practice of drying flowers for fragrances, decoration and as gifts dates back to the ancient Egyptians who placed dried flowers into tombs as gifts for the dead. In the Middle Ages, flowers were dried, crushed and used to ease ailments, including coughs, colds, toothaches, headaches and stomach pains.

Just because drying flowers is an ancient craft doesn't mean it's only for grannies. Potpourri and dried flower sachets make perfect, economical and thoughtful gifts. Here are a few simple tips to give it a modern-day twist.

Choosing and picking

Pardon the pun here, but when picking, you do need to be picky. Not all flowers are great for drying. For example, as beautiful as hydrangeas are, unless they are dried straight after picking using particular methods, they will lose their gorgeous pastel colours and become as brown as the dirt they came from. As a general rule, delicate flowers are a little harder to dry the old-fashioned way (in the sun), but most can be dried using a dehydrator (see page 58).

The whole point of making potpourri is to cover up bad smells with pretty floral ones. Unfortunately not all petals smell that pretty when they are dried out, so choose wisely: the more fragrant they are on the actual bush, the better they will smell in the bowl. Picked on a hot summer's day when the flowers are completely dry, tuberoses are perfect – just make sure they actually smell! Hybrid tea roses these days sometimes have no smell at all.

I like to use rice flowers, roses, dandelions, violets, lavender, cornflowers, nasturtiums, gerberas, snapdragons, poppies and sage leaves. I always include some flowers more for their looks than their scent, so that the finished mixture looks bright and textured. I also love the misty (available all year in Australia) or a David Austin in the UK.

Pick them when the petals are almost ready to fall off the receptacle (the part the petals are attached to). Before you pick the flower, give it a little shake so that any bugs hiding inside can find another place to stay.

Potpourri continued

Drying

Once picked, you can either use a dehydrator (see below) or dry the petals and leaves the old-fashioned way. To do this, put some sheets of kitchen paper on trays and lay out the petals separately, spreading them apart so the air can circulate. The paper helps to draw any moisture away from the petals. Find a place out of draughts to dry the petals, preferably inside. Near a window is good to give them sufficient sunlight for drying – direct sunlight dries them quicker but they fade a little too.

Leave them for 1–2 days. Check on them as they may dry quicker depending on your home: they like dry heat, no humidity. When they are ready, they feel like tissue paper and wrinkle up a little. Once they're done, I suggest putting them straight into an airtight container lined with kitchen paper until you are ready to use them.

To dehydrate your flowers, preheat the dehydrator to a low heat (between 35–45°C, although this will vary). Remember, the thicker the petal the higher the heat, so for delicate rose petals, for example, you may need to reduce the heat to about 30°C. As a general rule, if you live in a humid country, you can dehydrate at around 55°C. Cut any stems off the flowers. Before placing them in the dehydrator, shake off any critters from the flowers back into the garden – I'm not sure they would appreciate the sunburn! Check on your flowers every hour until they are fully dehydrated to your liking. As long as there is no moisture in the petal, your flower will last.

Making the potpourri

If you choose a strong-smelling flower, your potpourri should retain its scent for about 6 months, and you can then add essential oils as the smell dissipates. If not, you can use a fixative in the form of orris root powder or oakmoss (the instructions for this come with the product). The rest is up to you. Choose your mix of essential oils and add a few drops to your dried flower petals. Try to be sparing to start with, depending on how much mix you have, and then add more drops if necessary.

Place the mix into a pretty ball jar or tip into a linen bag and voilà, not so granny-like potpourri. I also love to fill a little ceramic or metal bowl with potpourri and place in guest rooms and the bathroom.

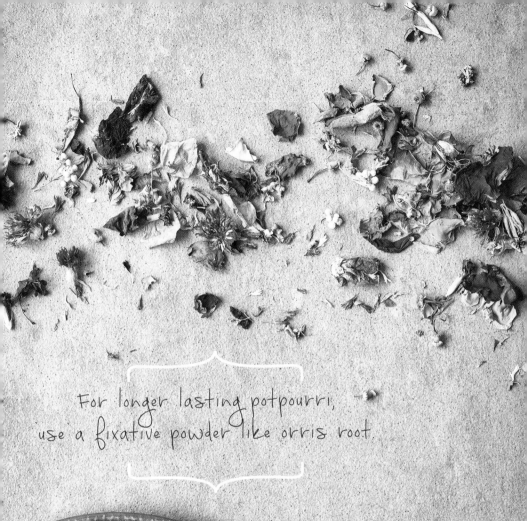

For longer lasting potpourri,
use a fixative powder like orris root.

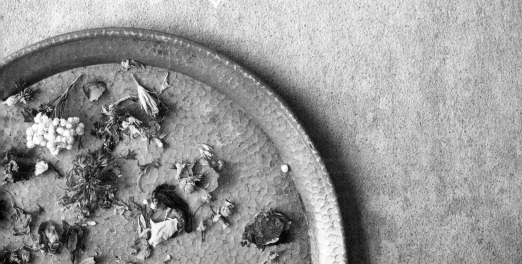

Coffee candles (to get rid of odours)

Coffee is by far one of the greatest smells in the world to me. It is comforting, invigorating and makes me salivate just a little. It's also fantastic for removing odours.

MAKES 1–2 CANDLES
(depending on the size of your moulds)

500g soy wax or paraffin wax, chopped or grated

1–2 tablespoons ground coffee

1 teaspoon whole coffee beans, plus extra to decorate the top (optional – they tend to crackle and pop as they heat up, so you may prefer to leave them out)

thermometer

candle moulds (anything from small glass jars, tins and pots)

spray oil

wicks

hairdryer

If you are using a double boiler, get it set up. If you don't have one, boil some water in a large saucepan, then turn the heat down so the water is barely simmering, and set a heatproof bowl on top of the saucepan (making sure the bottom of the bowl doesn't touch the water underneath). Add the wax to the top of the double boiler or to the bowl and leave to melt, stirring every so often. Use a thermometer to ensure the temperature of the wax does not exceed 90°C.

Add the ground coffee and coffee beans (if using) and stir in. Remove from the heat once the coffee has been added and mixed so that it is evenly distributed. Set aside and quickly prep your moulds.

Insert a wick into your mould by tying the wick to a pencil and sitting it horizontally across the top of the mould so that the wick hangs vertically. Carefully pour in the wax to about 2cm from the top, then leave to cool and set. The candle sometimes shrinks in the centre as it cools, so once it has set you can add a little more melted wax if needed. Use a hair dryer to dispel any air bubbles or divots, and smooth the top. Sprinkle a few more coffee beans over the top. Cut off the wick and then leave each candle for at least 24 hours before lighting it.

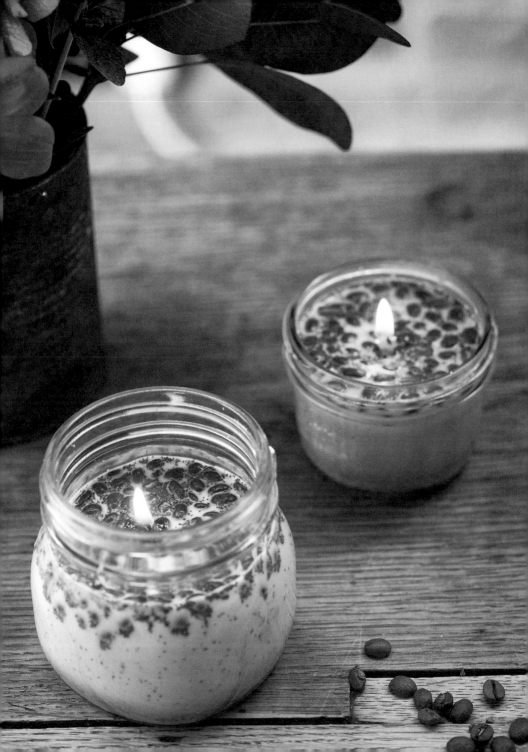

Room freshener two ways

When you don't have fresh flowers but you wish your house smelt like them, try making your own scented spray. Play around with the scents to your liking. Both of these air fresheners will keep for up to a year and you can use them as often as you like. Adding essential oils will give the smell more oomph and make them last a lot longer in the air so I highly recommend using them.

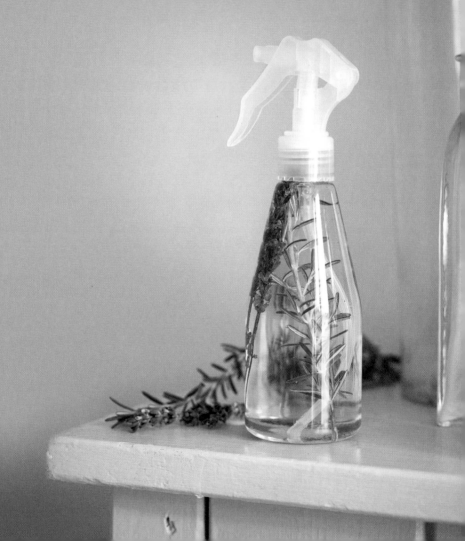

Rosemary, Sage & Lavender Air Freshener

This is an invigorating and floral air freshener – not sickly or fake-smelling, more like your nana's garden in spring. Rosemary and lavender go together perfectly.

MAKES 500ML

4 sprigs of rosemary

2 sprigs of sage

2 teaspoons dried lavender or
   3 sprigs of fresh lavender

2 lemon slices

500ml water

4 drops each of rosemary and
   lavender essential oils (not a
   must but these will give more
   oomph to the spray)

500ml spray bottle (recycled
   is fine)

Place all the ingredients in a small saucepan. Bring to a simmer over a medium heat, then cover and leave the mix to simmer for a further 5 minutes.

Remove from the heat and leave it to cool, then pour into a spray bottle – there's no need to strain the ingredients as they will continue to infuse in the bottle (though you can strain them out if you prefer). If the sprigs are too tall for the bottle, just break them in half; you can also twist the lemon slices and add them at the end, fresh, if you prefer.

Refresh the herbs and lemon slices in the bottle regularly to keep the smell lively, as it will dull over time. If they become mouldy, just remove and discard them. This will keep for up to a year and you can use it as often as needed.

Lemongrass, lime & ginger air Freshener

This one is a great pick-me-up air freshener that will give your home a clean, fresh, energising smell.

MAKES 500ML

2 limes, sliced

2 fresh lemongrass stalks, crushed a little

10cm piece of fresh ginger, crushed with a knife

500ml water

4 drops each of lemongrass and ginger essential oils (not a must but will give more oomph to the spray)

500ml spray bottle (recycled is fine)

Place all the ingredients in a small saucepan. Bring to a simmer over a medium heat, then cover and leave the mix to simmer for a further 5 minutes.

Remove from the heat and leave it to cool, then pour into a spray bottle – there's no need to strain the ingredients as they will continue to infuse in the bottle (though you can strain them out if you prefer). If the lemongrass stalks are too tall for the bottle, just break them in half; you can also twist the lime slices and add them at the end, fresh, if you prefer.

Refresh the spices and lime slices in the bottle often to keep the smell lively, as it will dull over time. If they become mouldy, just remove and discard them.

This will keep for up to a year and you can use it as often as needed.

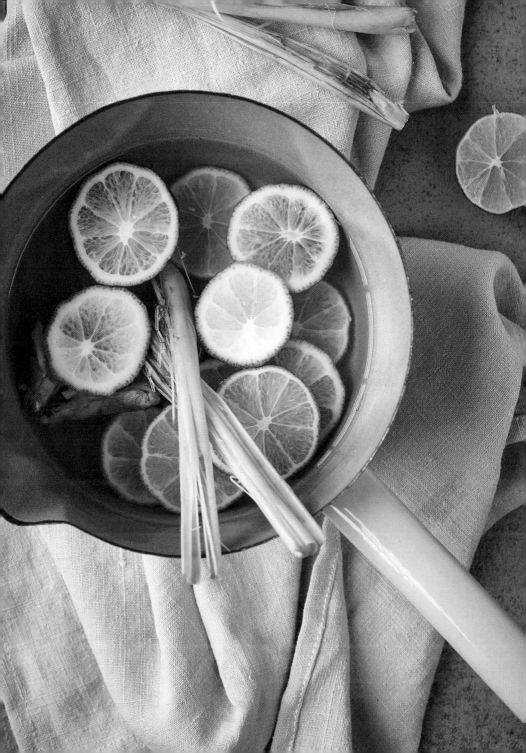

Chapter Five

make it shine

Wood polish

Here's a great polish to stop your wood from ageing and also to help spruce it up when it's looking tired. It works on dark wood best. Always test this on a small, inconspicuous area first to see how you like the post-polish look.

MAKES 225ML

3 tablespoons olive oil

180ml vinegar (use white vinegar for light wood and apple cider vinegar for dark wood)

30 drops of orange oil or pine oil, or a combination of both

1 spray bottle

Put everything in a spray bottle and shake to mix.

This will keep in the cupboard under the sink or in the laundry room for up to a year. When using, spray lightly on the surface and rub with a soft cloth to polish.

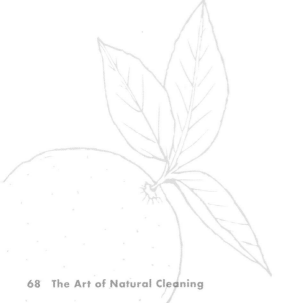

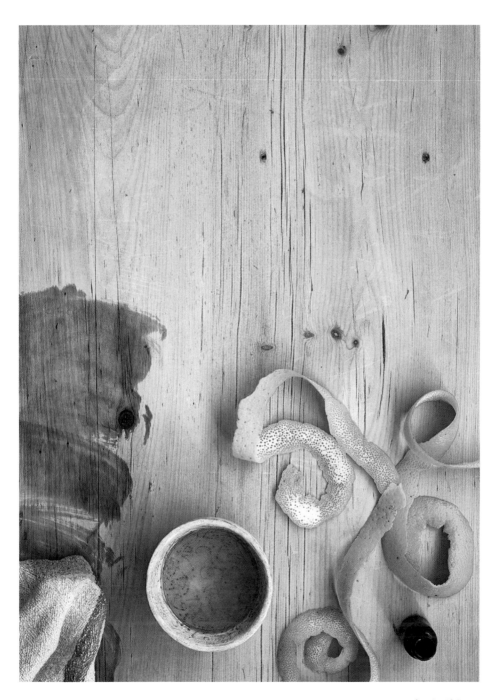

Mould no more

Mould is only good on cheese. Anywhere else (for example, mould in bathrooms from dampness or mould on carpets) and I would say it's best to wipe it away. Give this chemical-free spray a go. It has a strong smell for a couple or so days, but it beats the smell of mould, hands down..

MAKES 510ML

3 teaspoons tea tree essential oil

spray bottle

Combine the tea tree essential oil with 500ml water in a spray bottle and shake to blend. Spray onto problem areas, leave for 5 minutes, then wipe away the mould, but do not rinse off. This mixture will keep indefinitely, and you can use it as required.

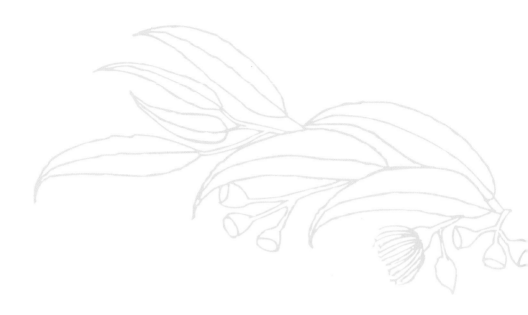

Floor cleaner

This is great for marble, ceramic, concrete, lino or tiled floors. Always sweep before mopping for best results. Turn up the tunes and drink the rest of the vodka as you mop, for even better results!

MAKES ENOUGH
FOR 1 APPLICATION

100ml white vinegar

50ml cheap vodka (high-proof is best)

5 drops of eucalyptus essential oil

5 drops of tea tree essential oil

1 teaspoon liquid castile soap

warm water, to top up

Place all the ingredients in a mop bucket, then top up with warm water. Stir well, then use it to mop your floors as normal. Leave to dry (no need to rinse).

For shiny brass

Have you ever noticed how much brass your gran has at home and how shiny it always is? This is how she keeps it that way!

MAKES ENOUGH
FOR 1 APPLICATION
juice of ½ small lemon
1 teaspoon bicarbonate of soda

Squeeze the lemon juice into a small bowl, then add the bicarbonate of soda and stir together to make a thin paste. Using a soft cloth, gently work the paste into the brass in one direction as best as possible. Rinse off with water and dry well.

Reapply and repeat the process until the brass is shiny. When you're satisfied, give the brass a rinse in water, making sure there's no paste left, then dry and polish it with a clean, dry soft cloth.

If you're not an expert, sometimes you may not realise what's brass and what's not. The easiest way to check is to hold a fridge magnet to it. If it sticks, it's not brass.

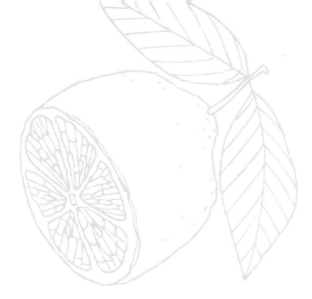

Window cleaner

Cleaning windows is a total drag, especially when all the efforts leave streaks anyway. Try this recipe, and for best results, rinse with water and use a squeegee for a final sparkle.

MAKES 635ML

125ml white vinegar
2 teaspoons liquid castile soap

spray bottle

Place all the vinegar and castile soap in a clean spray bottle with 500ml water and shake together until mixed. Spray onto windows, then scrub with sheets of crumpled newspaper or a soft cloth. Rinse with water and use a squeegee to remove the water.

This will keep for up to 3 months, and you can use it as required.

Resources

Below are just some of the fantastic suppliers you can source your ingredients and equipment from.

WORLDWIDE DELIVERY

New Directions
For cosmetic bases, essential oils, castile soap, bottles and jars, packaging and dried ingredients
www.newdirections.com.au

Amazon
For cosmetic bases, essential oils, carrier oils, castile soap, bottles and jars, packaging and dried ingredients
www.amazon.co.uk or
www.amazon.com

Bulk Apothecary
For cosmetic bases, essential oils, castile soap, bottles and jars, packaging and dried ingredients
www.bulkapothecary.com

Baldwins
For cosmetic bases, essential oils, castile soap, bottles and jars, packaging and dried ingredients
www.baldwins.co.uk

Wholesale Mineral Makeup
For mica and make up ingredients, with worlwide delivery
www.wholesalemineralmakeup.com.au

Speciality Bottle
Bottles and cosmetic equipment
www.specialtybottle.com

Organic alcohol
Alcohol for cleaning
www.organicalcohol.com

UK

Neal's Yard
For dried herbs, essential oils and carrier oils
www.nealsyardremedies.com

Pestle Herbs
For fried Herbs and apothecary bottles
www.pestleherbs.co.uk

AUSTRALIA

Austral Herbs
For dried herbs and flowers
www.australherbs.com.au

Essentially Australia
For essential oils
www. essentiallyaustralia.com.au

USA & CANADA

Mountain Rose Herbs
For dried herbs and flowers
www.mountainroseherbs.com

Index

Index continued

P

pans, cleaning burnt 24

peppermint

  moth balls 28

petals

  drawer liners 32

  linen sachets 30

  potpourri 57–9

  toilet bombs 44

pine

  herby floral burn sticks 54

pine essential oil

  wood polish 68

polishes 67–73

  brass polish 72

  floor cleaner 70

  shoe polish 34

  window cleaner 73

  wood polish 68

potpourri 57–9

R

room fresheners 62–4

rose essential oil

  toilet bombs 44

rose petals

  linen sachets 30

rose twigs

  herby floral burn sticks 54

rosemary

  herby floral burn sticks 54

moth balls 28

rosemary, sage & lavender air freshener 63

rubbish bins, odour eaters 50

S

sage

  herby floral burn sticks 54

  rosemary, sage & lavender air freshener 63

salt 8

  cleaning wooden chopping boards 22

  dishwasher detergent 21

  odour eaters 50

  salt scourer 14

scent 49–65

  coffee candles 60

  diffusers 52

  herby floral burn sticks 54

  odour eaters 50

  potpourri 57–9

  room fresheners 62–4

scourer, salt 14

shoes

  odour eaters 50

  shoe polish 34

sinks, odour eaters 50

soap (liquid castile) 8

  floor cleaner 70

  hand wash 20

  washing powder 37

  washing-up liquid 19

  window cleaner 73

soda (washing)

  washing powder 37

sofas, odour eaters 50

T

tea tree essential oil

  anti-bacterial wipes 46

  floor cleaner 70

  mould remover 71

toilets

  odour eaters 50

  toilet bombs 44

U

upholstery, odour eaters 50

V

vinegar 8

  anti-bacterial wipes 46

  bathroom cleaner 43

  cleaning burnt pans 24

  dishwasher detergent 21

  fabric softener 37

  floor cleaner 70

  orange all-round kitchen spray 12

  oven cleaner 17

Acknowledgements

Firstly to my family. My mum and dad have always supported me and I love that they sit in what my dad calls his 'proud chair' because of the path I am on. All I have ever wanted was to make them and my brothers proud. So to you my small family and the rest of my big extended family, especially its oh so wonderful leader my nan (and great grandmother Lil). To all of you, Sarah, Nigel, Paul, Mark, Kylie, Skye, Angie, Bec, Harry, Nicole, Yasmin, Sam, Teryn, Ashleigh, Caitlyn, Liam, Brad and Taylah and then the rest of our little family Emma, Koen and my godsons Charlie and Rory. You are all everything to me. As are you Damien, my love. Thank you for putting up with our home looking like a constant laboratory and test kitchen. To my friends who have supported me for decades. To Kyle. I have no words to express how grateful I am to you. To our new Octopus family, here is to a long journey making beautiful and meaningful books together. To my team. The A team. Tara, the most incredible Editor a girl could ask for. Your patience, generosity and passion for these next books made them what they are. Nassima. Thank you for making my recipes and creations come to life. I only hope we work on many a more things together. Rachel. No words can thank you enough for being the most incredible partner in crime styling these books and seeing inside my messy brain. You are so immensely talented and I am so grateful. Agathe, Laura and the rest of the team. High fives all round! To all of the people in my work world who have taught me so very much over the years. Thank you. There is no way I would be where I am without you teaching me everything I know. Last but not at all least, to all of you who bought this book. Massive gratitude from the bottom of my heart.

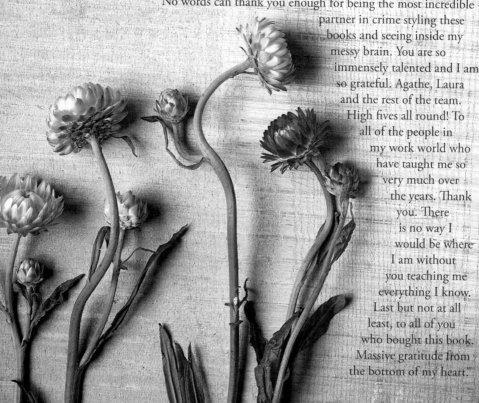